SUZANNE WOODS

Healing in Nature

Embracing Ecotherapy to Heal Body, Mind and Spirit

For my children and grandchildren

"Hold on to what is good, Even if it's a handful of earth. Hold on to what you believe, Even if it's a tree that stands by itself. Hold on to what you must do, Even if it's a long way from here. Hold on to your life, Even if it's easier to let go. Hold on to my hand, Even if someday I'll be gone away from you."
— Chief Crowfoot, Blackfoot

Contents

Introduction

"Nature itself is the best physician." Hippocrates

Welcome to '**Healing in Nature: Embracing Ecotherapy to Heal Body, Mind and Spirit',** your guide to understanding and experiencing the profound benefits of ecotherapy.

Ecotherapy, also known as nature therapy or green therapy, is a practice that helps individuals reconnect with the natural world to enhance physical, mental, and emotional well-being. It incorporates various outdoor activities and experiences that promote healing and balance.

Historically, humans have always had a deep bond with nature, relying on it not only for sustenance but also for healing and spiritual rejuvenation. In recent years, with the rise of urbanization and the stressors of modern life, the importance of reconnecting with nature has become more evident.

Numerous scientific studies have shown that spending time in natural settings can lead to significant improvements in mood, stress levels, and overall health. This book will take you on a journey through the many facets of ecotherapy, from the foundational principles to practical applications.

We'll explore different forms of ecotherapy, such as forest bathing, gardening, water therapy, grounding, wilderness therapy and animal-assisted therapy, and delve into their unique benefits. Whether you are new to the concept or looking to deepen your understanding, this book will provide you with the knowledge and tools to harness the healing power of nature.

So, take a deep breath, imagine the fresh scent of pine trees or the soothing sound of flowing water, and let's embark on this adventure together!

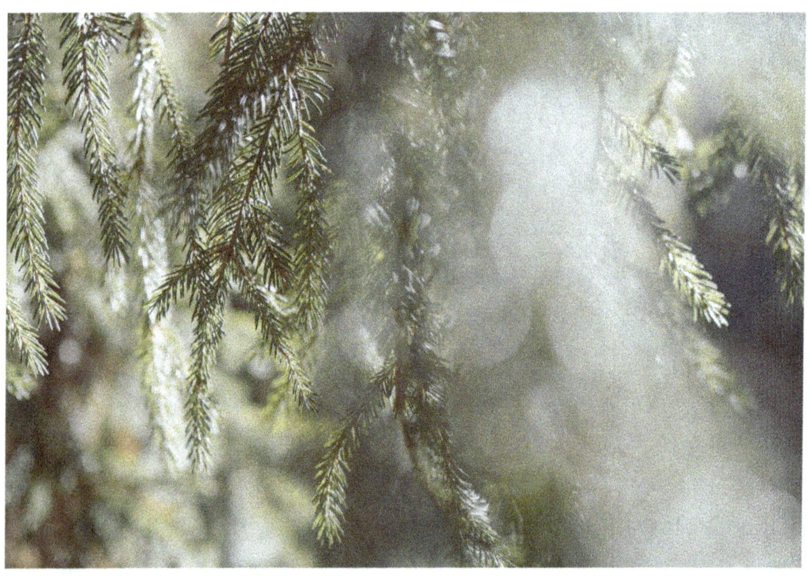

1

What is Ecotherapy?

"Look deep into nature, and then you will understand everything better" – Albert Einstein.

Ecotherapy, also known as nature therapy, is a practice that falls under the broader category of therapeutic approaches which emphasize the importance of the natural environment in mental and physical health. At its core, ecotherapy revolves around the simple yet profound concept that nature has a healing effect on us. Ecotherapy involves participating in various nature-based activities, like gardening, walking in the park, or even engaging in more specialized practices, such as forest bathing and wilderness therapy, to promote well-being and reduce stress and anxiety.

The term 'ecotherapy' is relatively modern, gaining popularity in the late 20th and early 21st centuries. However, its roots can be traced back to ancient civilizations that recognized and revered the healing power of nature. Indigenous cultures across the globe have long practised nature-based healing, using the natural world as medicine and a means to restore balance.

One of the critical principles of ecotherapy is the connection between human beings and the natural environment. Nature provides us with shelter, food, and other essentials for survival. It also nourishes our mental and emotional well-being. In modern times, with an increasing emphasis on technology and urbanization, many people have become disconnected from nature, leading to an array of health issues such as anxiety, depression, and a sense of isolation. Ecotherapy seeks to bridge this gap and reconnect individuals with the natural world.

"The old Lakota was wise. He knew that a man's heart away from nature becomes hard. He knew that lack of respect for growing, living things soon led to lack of respect for humans, too. So he kept his children close to nature's softening influence."
Luther Standing Bear (Chief) 1868 – 1939
Oglala Lakota

Several scientific studies substantiate the efficacy of ecotherapy. Research has shown that spending time in green spaces can lower blood pressure, reduce cortisol levels (a stress hormone), and enhance cognitive function. Additionally, exposure to natural light and fresh air has been linked to improved mood and mental clarity. By integrating nature into therapeutic practices, ecotherapy can help individuals achieve greater peace and well-being.

There are various forms of ecotherapy, each tailored to different interests and needs. Some of the most common forms include:

1. **Nature Walks and Hikes**: Simply walking in a park, forest, or along a beach can be incredibly therapeutic. The sensory experience of hearing birds chirp, feeling the breeze, and observing the greenery can work wonders for mental health.

2. **Gardening**: Gardening activities can be both relaxing and rewarding. Digging in the soil, planting seeds, and nurturing plants to grow can provide a sense of accomplishment and grounding.

3. **Forest Bathing** (Shinrin-yoku): Originating in Japan, forest bathing involves immersing oneself in a forest environment to promote relaxation and reduce stress. This practice emphasizes mindfulness and sensory awareness.

4. **Animal-Assisted Ecotherapy**: Interaction with animals, such as therapy dogs, horses, or even dolphins, can have calming and positive effects on mental health. Animals can offer comfort, reduce loneliness, and improve social interaction.

5. **Water Therapy**: Spending time near bodies of water, whether a lake, river or ocean, has been shown to reduce stress and promote tranquility. Activities such as swimming, fishing, or simply sitting by the water can be very calming.

By understanding and embracing the various forms of ecotherapy, individuals can find the approach that resonates best with them and incorporate it into their daily routines. The beauty of ecotherapy lies in its versatility and accessibility; regardless of where you live or your level of familiarity with nature, there is always a way to experience the healing power of the natural world.

2

The Healing Power of Green Spaces

"We must protect the forests for our children, grandchildren and children yet to be born. We must protect the forests for those who can't speak for themselves such as the birds, animals, fish and trees."

– Qwatsinas (Hereditary Chief Edward Moody), Nuxalk Nation

In our busy lives, it's easy to forget the simple joys that nature brings. Green spaces, whether expansive forests, city parks, or humble backyard gardens, have an incredible power to heal our bodies and minds. Here, we investigate why these green oases are more than just a pleasing escape—they are essential for our well-being.

Why are forests so important?

Forests of all sizes play an essential role in the health of the Earth, acting as the Earth's "lungs". Trees and plants absorb the carbon dioxide we breathe out and, through photosynthesis, produce oxygen, which is essential to us. Trees also trap harmful pollutants in their leaves and branches, acting as an air filter to give us cleaner air to breathe.

Forests are home to more than half of the world's land-based animals, plants, and insects. These species interact with each other, each playing a crucial role in supporting all life on this planet. As each species of animal or plant disappears, life on Earth becomes more unstable and uninhabitable. Biodiversity, the variety of living things on our planet, is vital for all life on Earth.

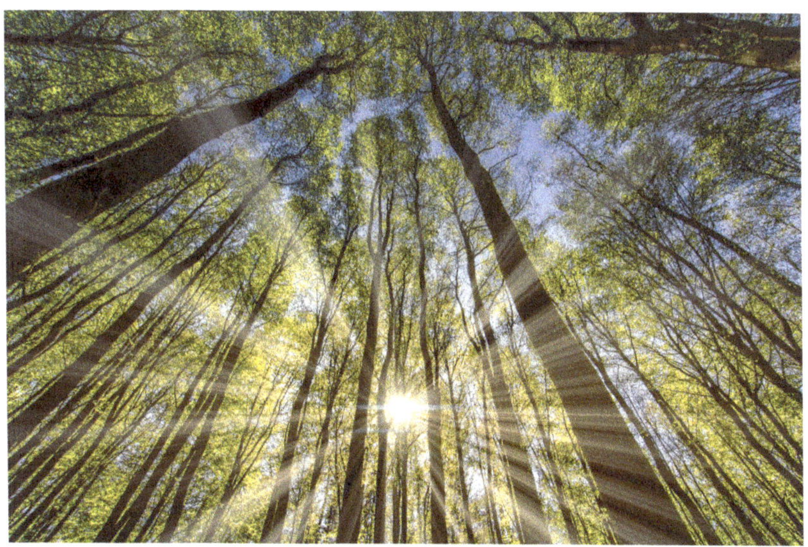

Spending time in green spaces has many **physical benefits**; for example, it has been shown to lower blood pressure, reduce the risk of heart disease, and improve overall fitness levels. Walking through a park or hiking a forest trail, you're not just enjoying the scenery; you're giving your body a gentle workout. Your muscles engage, your lungs fill with fresh air, and your heart pumps with a joyous rhythm. One study found that spending just 120 minutes a week in nature significantly boosts overall health and well-being.

However, the magic of green spaces goes beyond physical health. Time spent in nature has profound **mental health benefits** as well. Have you ever noticed how a walk in the park can clear your mind and lift your spirits? That's because green spaces help reduce stress and anxiety. Nature has a soothing effect on our minds, lowering cortisol levels and banishing the mental fatigue that modern life brings. A stroll among the trees can rejuvenate your mental state, helping you feel more relaxed and focused.

As for **cognitive benefits**, nature can enhance creativity and improve concentration. Many artists and writers have found inspiration in the great outdoors. Studies suggest that even short periods spent in nature can enhance problem-solving skills and boost creativity. So, the next time you're stuck on a challenging project or need a fresh burst of ideas, consider taking a break and heading to the nearest park.

While personal anecdotal evidence is compelling, **scientific research** backs up these claims. For instance, a study conducted by the University of Exeter found that people who live in urban areas with more green space have greater well-being and lower levels of mental distress. Another study by Stanford University highlighted how nature experiences reduce rumination, a maladaptive pattern of self-referential thought that is linked to mental illnesses such as depression and anxiety.

Green spaces also **foster social connections**. Parks and community gardens are often bustling with people engaging in friendly conversations, playing sports, or simply enjoying the scenery. These interactions help combat loneliness and build a sense of belonging. Research shows that people who spend more time in green spaces tend to have stronger social ties and higher levels of community engagement.

In essence, green spaces offer a multifaceted approach to healing. They cater to our physical needs, nurture our mental well-being, enhance our cognitive abilities, and foster social interactions. As urbanization continues to rise, integrating more green spaces into our environments becomes crucial. These areas serve as sanctuaries where we can reconnect with nature, find balance, and rejuvenate our spirits.

So, the next time you feel overwhelmed or need a break from the daily grind, step into a green space. Your body, mind, and spirit will thank you. Embrace nature's healing power and let it work its magic. Sometimes, the best medicine really is a walk in the park.

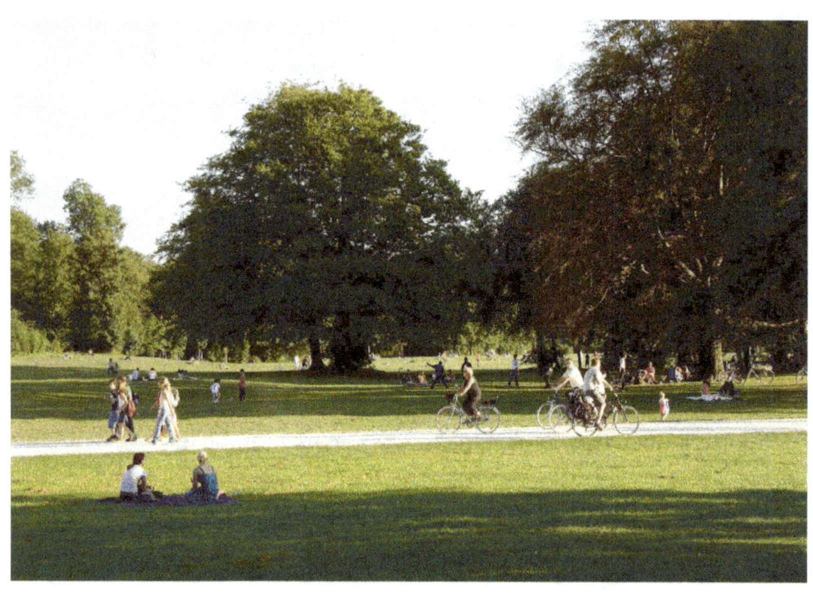

3

Forest Bathing: Shinrin-yoku

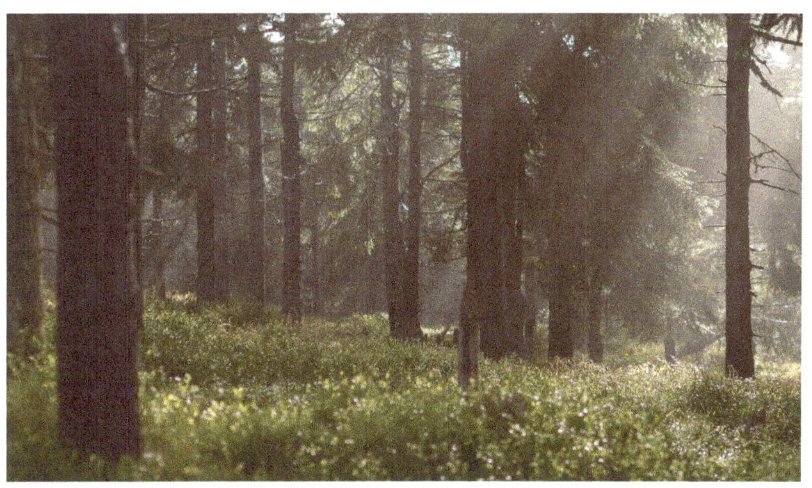

"And into the forest I go to lose my mind and find my soul."– John Muir

Forest Bathing, known as Shinrin-yoku, is a Japanese practice that involves immersing oneself in a forest environment to promote mental and physical well-being. The term 'Shinrin-yoku' directly translates to 'forest bath,' and it was developed in Japan during the 1980s to counteract the increasing stress and tech-driven lifestyles people were experiencing. This practice has since gained popularity worldwide as nature lovers and wellness enthusiasts recognize the profound benefits of spending time among the trees.

The idea behind forest bathing is simple: take a slow, mindful walk through the forest, engaging all your senses to experience the natural surroundings fully. Unlike hiking, which often focuses on reaching a destination, forest bathing emphasizes the journey, encouraging participants to move slowly, breathe deeply, and become aware of the sights, sounds, and scents around them. The key is to be present in the moment and to absorb the tranquility of the forest environment.

Scientific research backs the health benefits of Shinrin-yoku. Studies have shown that spending time in nature, particularly in forested areas, can reduce stress, lower blood pressure, improve mood, boost immune system function, and increase overall well-being. One way forest bathing achieves these effects is through the inhalation of phytoncides, natural compounds released by trees and plants that have antimicrobial properties. Phytoncides not only help plants protect themselves from harmful organisms, but they also offer health benefits to humans who breathe them in.

Forest bathing also promotes mindfulness, which has been linked to numerous psychological benefits, including reduced anxiety and depression, improved attention and concentration, and enhanced creativity. When you intentionally slow down and engage with the forest using all your senses, you cultivate a mindful state that allows you to disconnect from daily stressors and reconnect with your inner self.

Forest bathing is accessible to anyone, regardless of fitness level or location. You don't need to trek deep into a remote wilderness; a local park or nearby woods can provide a suitable setting. To get started with forest bathing, follow these simple steps:

1. Choose a forest or wooded area where you feel safe and comfortable. This could be a nearby national park, a nature reserve, or even a well-wooded urban park.

2. Leave behind your electronic devices or set them to silent mode to minimize distractions. The goal is to disconnect from technology and reconnect with nature.

3. As you enter the forest, take a few deep breaths and set an intention to explore the environment with all your senses mindfully.

4. Begin your walk slowly, paying attention to the sights, sounds, smells, and textures around you. Notice the rustling leaves, the chirping of birds, the earthy scent of the forest floor, and the feeling of the ground beneath your feet.

5. If you come across a spot that particularly draws your attention, feel free to sit or stand there for a while, simply observing and soaking in the atmosphere.

6. Continue at your own pace, allowing yourself to be fully present and open to whatever the forest offers. Permitting your mind to wander and thoughts to arise naturally is part of the process.

7. When you feel ready, slowly make your way back to where you started, again savouring each step and sensory experience along the way.

Incorporating regular forest bathing sessions into your routine can have lasting positive effects on your mental and physical health. By making a conscious effort to spend time in nature, you can create a sanctuary of calm and rejuvenation within your daily life.

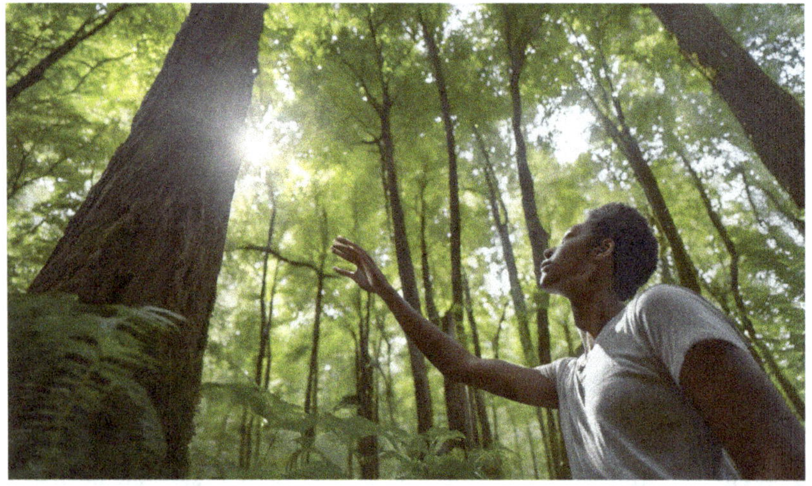

Be safe: If you are going alone, tell someone where you are going, go to a place where you will be safe, and do not stray from the path, to avoid getting lost.

4

15

Gardening as Therapy

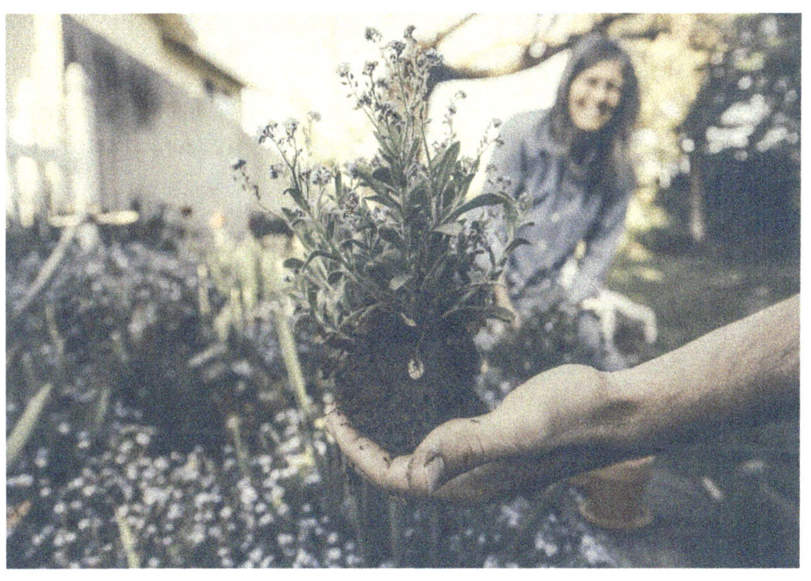

Gardening is more than just a pastime; it's a therapeutic activity proven to provide mental, physical, and emotional benefits. For centuries, humans have been cultivating plants, finding solace and meaning in the simple act of tending to a garden. This chapter explores the therapeutic benefits of gardening, the different types of healing gardens, and offers practical tips for starting your own garden wherever you are.

The Therapeutic Benefits of Gardening

Gardening involves many activities, from planting and nurturing seeds to harvesting the fruits, vegetables, or flowers they produce. This hands-on engagement with nature promotes physical exercise, mental clarity, and emotional resilience. Here's how:

1. **Physical Health Benefits**: Gardening is a low-impact exercise that improves cardiovascular health, enhances flexibility, and strengthens muscles. From digging and planting to weeding and watering, the physical tasks involved in gardening help burn calories and build stamina. Regular interaction with soil has also been shown to bolster the immune system, with beneficial microbes found in soil potentially contributing to a healthy gut microbiome.

2. **Mental Health Benefits**: Connecting with nature through gardening can significantly reduce stress and anxiety. The rhythmic activity of digging, planting, and watering can be meditative and calming, providing a mental break from daily stresses. Many studies have indicated that spending time in green spaces lowers cortisol levels and boosts mood. Gardening also provides a sense of accomplishment and

purpose, particularly when plants start to thrive and bloom.

3. **Emotional Benefits**: Gardening offers a sense of responsibility and nurturing, which can be especially therapeutic for those dealing with grief or depression. It also fosters creativity and provides a way to express oneself through the design and care of the garden. Growing and sustaining life in a garden can be incredibly uplifting and affirming.

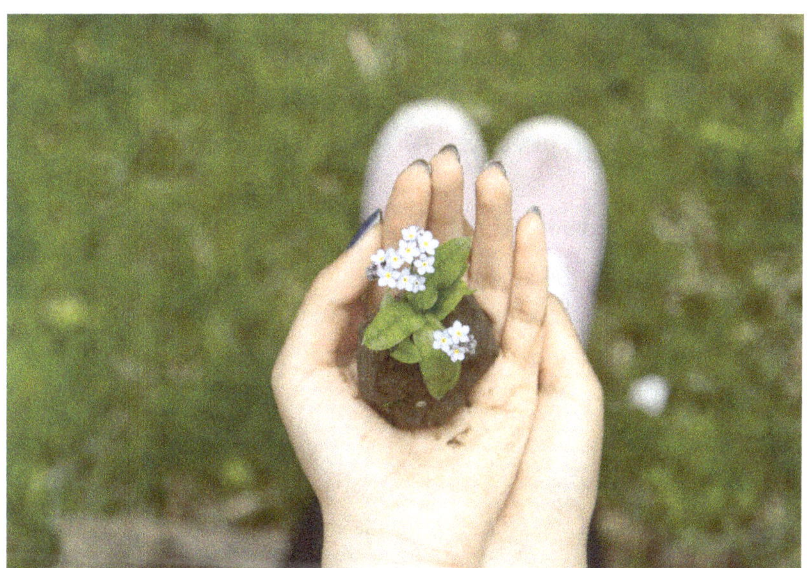

Healing Gardens

Healing gardens vary widely in form and function, but they all aim to promote health and well-being. Some popular types include:

1. **Therapeutic Horticulture Gardens**: These gardens are often used in healthcare settings as part of rehabilitation programs. They are designed to be accessible to everyone, including those with physical limitations, and include raised beds and wide pathways.

2. **Sensory Gardens**: These gardens are designed to stimulate all five senses. With fragrant flowers, textured plants, and soothing water features, they provide a whole sensory experience that can be especially beneficial for people with sensory processing disorders or dementia.

3. **Community Gardens**: These gardens bring people together, fostering social connections and a sense of community. They provide a shared space where people can grow vegetables, fruits, and flowers collectively, learning from one another and enjoying the companionship that gardening can bring.

4. **Meditation Gardens**: These gardens are designed to provide a peaceful, reflective space. They often include elements like zen gardens, water features, and quiet seating areas where individuals can meditate, pray, or simply relax.

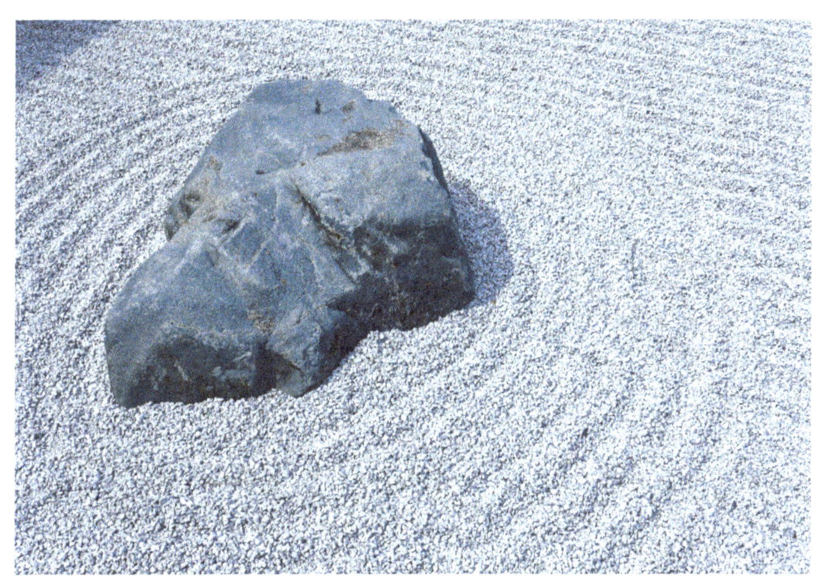

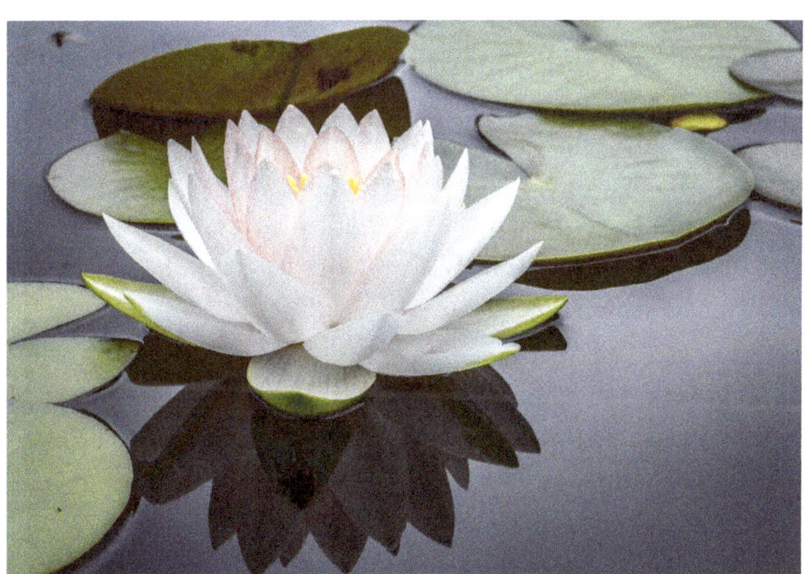

Starting Your Own Garden

Whether you have a large outdoor space or a small balcony, there are numerous possibilities for creating your garden. Here are some tips to get you started:

1. **Start Small**: If you're new to gardening, begin with a small plot or a few containers. This allows you to manage your garden without feeling overwhelmed.

2. **Choose the Right Plants**: Select plants that are well-suited to your climate and soil. Native plants are the best choice because they are adapted to the local environment and require less maintenance.

3. **Use Quality Soil**: Invest in good quality soil and compost. Healthy soil is the foundation of a successful garden, providing essential nutrients to your plants.

4. **Water Wisely**: Water your plants according to their needs. Overwatering can be as detrimental as underwatering. Pay attention to the moisture levels in the soil and avoid watering during the heat of the day to prevent evaporation.

5. **Be Patient**: Gardening is a gradual process. Enjoy the journey of watching your plants grow and develop. Remember that every challenge is an opportunity to learn and improve.

Gardening as therapy is accessible to everyone, regardless of age or experience. By incorporating the abovementioned practices, you can create a personal sanctuary that promotes health, happiness, and well-being. As you dig your hands into the earth, it's not just the plants that grow, but your sense of peace and connection to the natural world that flourishes.

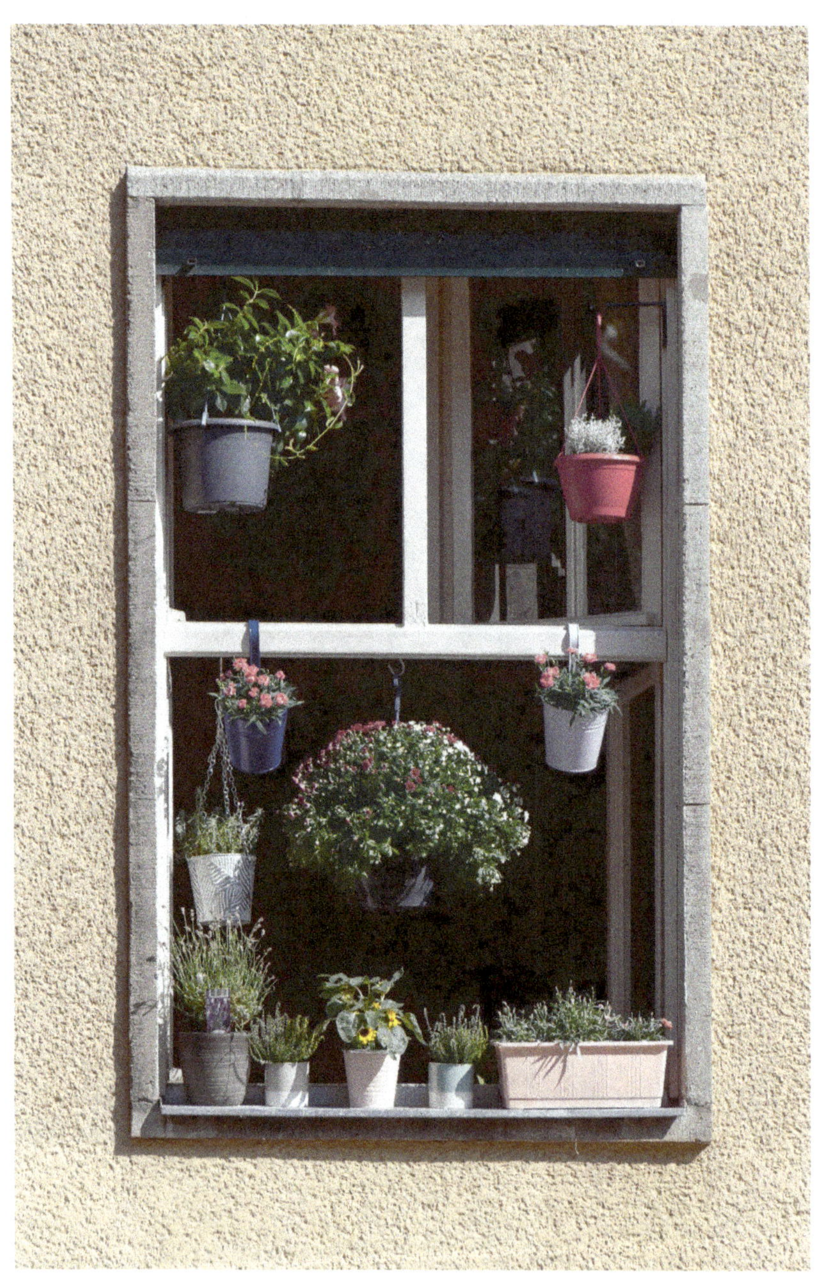

23

5

Water Therapy: The Magic of Blue Spaces

"I go to nature to be soothed and healed, and to have my senses put in order."
John Burroughs

The calming, restorative, and invigorating effects of water have been recognized for centuries. Ancient civilizations built their cities around rivers, springs, and oceans, understanding intuitively what modern science has confirmed: water has a profound impact on our health and well-being. This chapter delves into the fascinating world of water therapy, exploring how engaging with 'blue spaces' can bring serenity and healing into our lives.

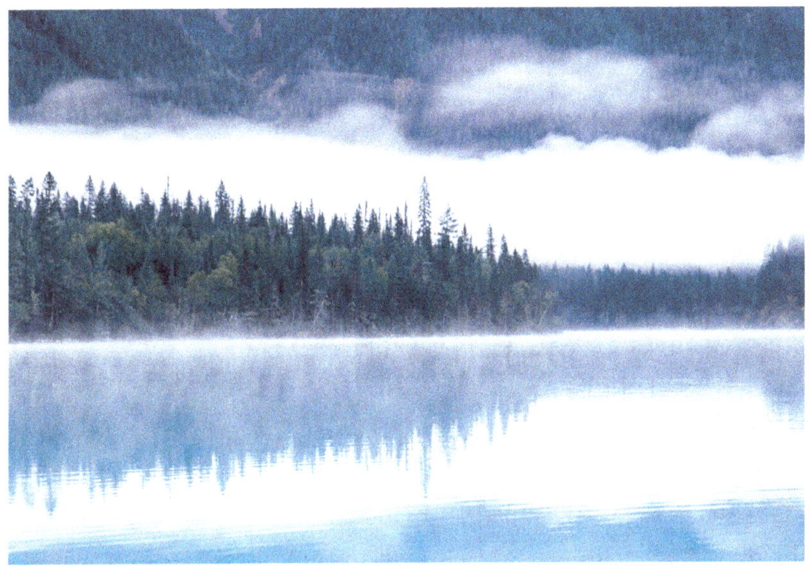

The Science Behind Water's Calming Effect

Water therapy, also known as hydrotherapy, encompasses a range of treatments involving water in different forms and settings. The underlying concept is simple but powerful: water has the ability to soothe stress, reduce anxiety, and promote mental clarity. Research has shown that being near water can lower blood pressure, decrease heart rate, and reduce levels of cortisol, the stress hormone. This is due to the unique way our brains and bodies respond to water environments.

One key element is the sound of water. The rhythmic sound of waves crashing, the gentle babbling of a brook, or the steady flow of a river are all 'non-threatening' sounds that help to soothe the autonomic nervous system. This system controls basic bodily functions such as heart rate and blood pressure. By calming this system, water sounds promote a meditative state, reducing stress and enhancing feelings of well-being.

Activities Involving Water Therapy

There are many ways to incorporate water therapy activities into your life, each offering its own set of benefits.

Swimming is not just a great workout; it's also an excellent way to relieve stress. The buoyancy of water supports your body, reducing the strain on joints and muscles. The repetitive motions of swimming, combined with the rhythmic breathing patterns, help create a meditative experience.

Fishing: Many find the simple act of sitting by a body of water, waiting for a bite, to be incredibly peaceful. Fishing requires patience and presence, which can help to take your mind off daily stresses and encourage mindfulness.

Kayaking and Canoeing: These activities combine physical exercise with the calming influence of water. Paddling through serene waters can provide a sense of adventure and freedom while allowing quiet introspection.

Incorporating Water Therapy Into Daily Life

You don't need to live by an ocean or lake to benefit from water therapy. Here are some practical ways to integrate it into your routine:

Baths and Showers: Transform your bath or shower time into a therapeutic ritual. The feel and sound of water can promote relaxation, relieve stress and anxiety, clear your mind, and even help you generate new ideas. Use this time to relax and let go of daily stresses entirely. You may like to add calming essential oils like lavender to your bathwater or use fragrant shower products.

Mini Fountains: Small indoor fountains can bring the sounds of water into your home or office. The gentle, trickling sound can create a calming atmosphere, helping you to focus and relax.

Visits to Local Water Bodies: Visit nearby lakes, rivers, or ponds regularly. Even a short walk by a water body can lower stress levels and improve your mood.

Case Studies and Personal Testimonials

The power of water therapy is not just theoretical; countless individuals have benefited from integrating blue spaces into their lives. Consider Jane, a high-stress corporate executive who found solace in evening kayak trips on a nearby lake. Over time, she noticed her anxiety levels drop, and her sleep quality improve. Then there's Mark, an overworked teacher who discovered the stimulating effects of swimming laps every morning. He credits this routine with giving him the mental clarity and energy to manage his classroom better.

Conclusion

Water therapy is a natural, accessible way to enhance your well-being. Whether swimming, fishing or simply sitting by the water's edge, incorporating blue spaces into your life can provide significant mental and physical health benefits. So, next time you're feeling stressed or overwhelmed, consider spending time near a body of water. You might find it's just what you need to restore your balance and tranquility.

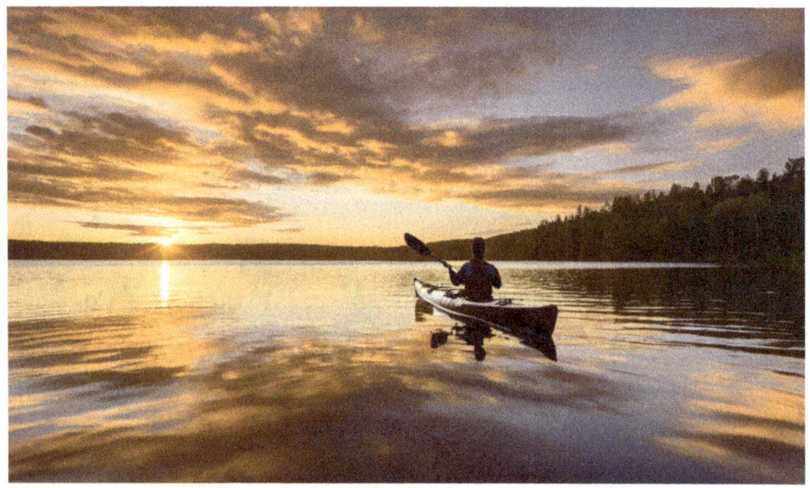

6

Sunsets, Beaches, Mountains and Flowers

"Just living is not enough... one must have sunshine, freedom, and a little flower."

Hans Christian Andersen

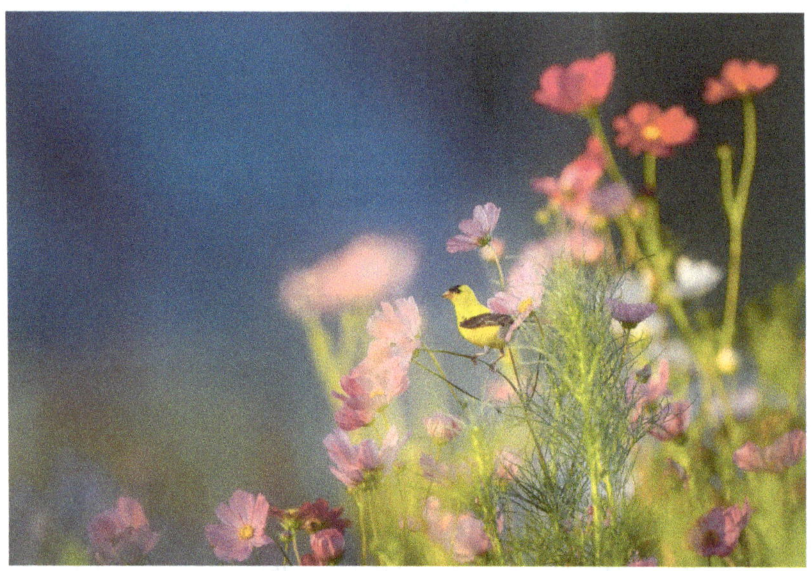

Colours of Nature

We have been emphasizing the calming green and blue of nature, which tend to dominate natural landscapes, but how about the other colours that can come into play in a natural scene? The warm reds, oranges and pinks in a sunset or autumn leaves; the earthy browns of a sandy beach; the bright white of a mountain covered in snow, or a rainbow in the sky, dazzling us with the whole spectrum of colours! Each colour has a particular effect on our minds, emotions, and bodies.

Colour Therapy, or Chromotherapy, has been used for thousands of years. It uses the colour energy of light. Natural light from the sun in itself is essential for our life and health. Each colour of the spectrum is simply light of a different wavelength. Thus, each colour has its own particular energy. Each colour, red, orange, yellow, green, blue, indigo, or violet, is said to resonate with one of the seven Chakras in our body's energy system. Colour can have a profound healing effect on us.

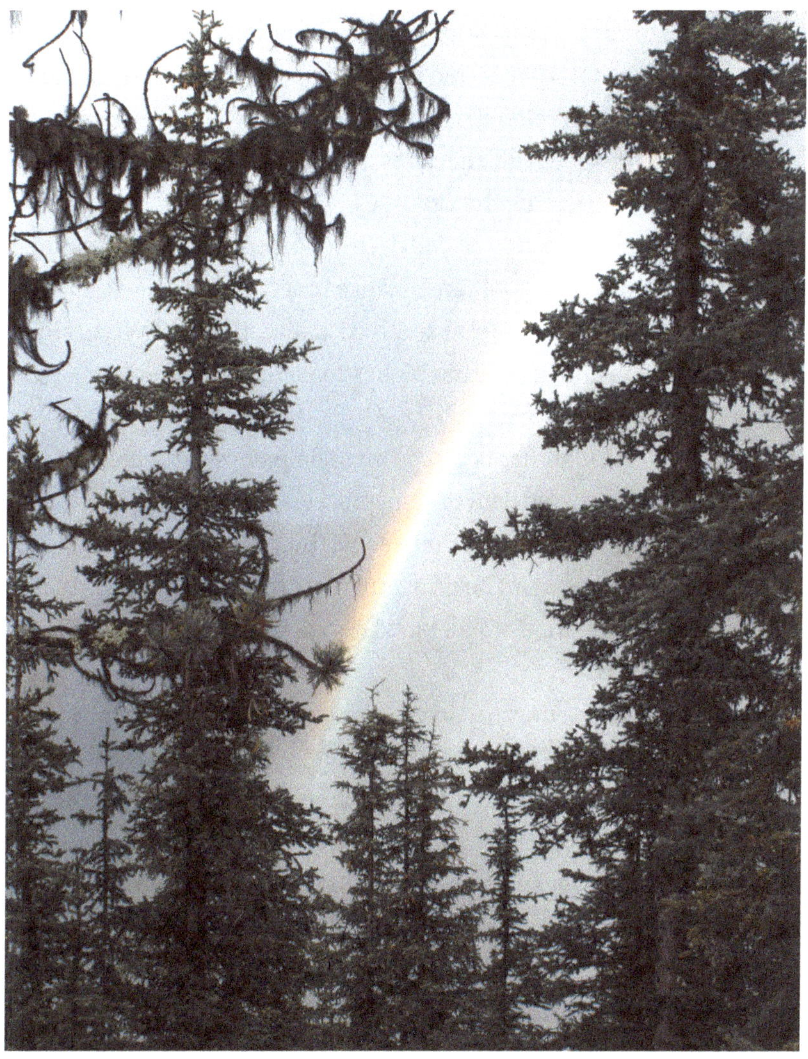

Red: Stimulates energy, vitality, and passion. It can enhance circulation and combat fatigue.

Orange: Promotes creativity and joy, aiding in emotional healing. It can boost enthusiasm and social interactions. It is used to stimulate the immune system, and treat depression and lack of motivation.

Yellow: Enhances mental clarity and focus, fostering optimism. It is also believed to support digestion and boost confidence.

Green: Represents balance and harmony, promoting relaxation and healing. It is often associated with physical healing and stress relief.

Blue: Calms the mind and alleviates anxiety. It is linked to communication and can help soothe throat issues.

Indigo: Encourages intuition and deep concentration. It is associated with spiritual awareness and can enhance inner peace.

Violet: Stimulates inspiration and spirituality. It is believed to aid in overcoming fears and promoting higher consciousness.

Red light, in particular, has been shown to help physical healing. It can reduce inflammation and pain in skin, muscles, and other tissues and is used in therapy to speed up wound healing by boosting circulation and allowing more oxygen and healing nutrients to reach the area. It also encourages the formation of new blood vessels and tissues and improves collagen levels.

Since red light, having the longest wavelength, can reach tissues below the skin's surface, it can penetrate the head into the brain. It has been shown to be good for learning, memory, reaction times and a positive mood. It may also be used to treat traumatic brain injuries and neurodegenerative conditions like dementia. Research is continuing to demonstrate the benefits of using red light therapy for stroke, depression, anxiety and other brain conditions, as well as dementia.

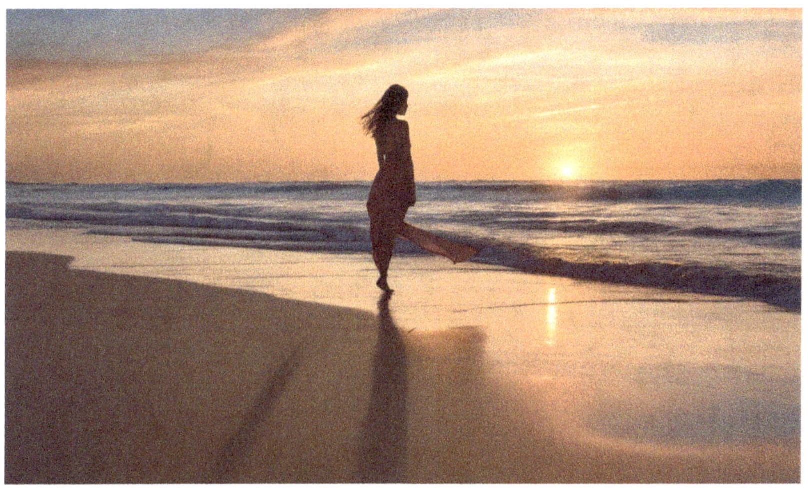

Awe-inspiring Nature

People find sunrises and sunsets to be the most beautiful and awe-inspiring weather, according to a study published in 2023 from the University of Exeter. This feeling of awe can improve mood, increase positive emotions, and decrease stress. "When you see something vast and overwhelming or something that produces this feeling of awe, your problems can feel diminished," the lead researcher says.

The feeling of awe may also be experienced in many other situations in nature: a view of mountains reaching high into the clouds, beautiful beaches stretching into the distance, or even the delicate petals of a small flower.

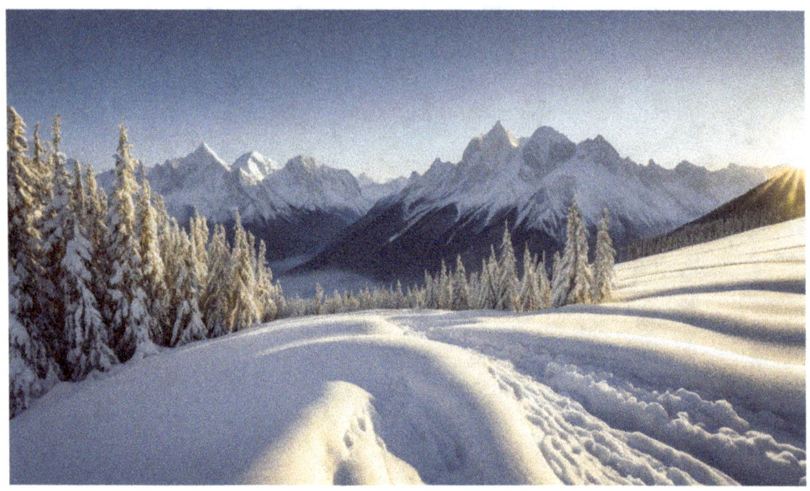

Do you need more reasons to go out into nature to appreciate its wonder and receive its healing? Even if you don't have a beach or beautiful scenery nearby, you can look up to the sky to see the clouds, stars, sunrise or sunset, or you may come across a pretty flower by the path on your walk. When you are aware of the many ways that nature can heal, you will begin to notice and appreciate what it presents.

"May the stars carry your sadness away, May the flowers fill your heart with beauty, May hope forever wipe away your tears, And, above all, may silence make you strong."
- Chief Dan George, Tsleil-Waututh Nation

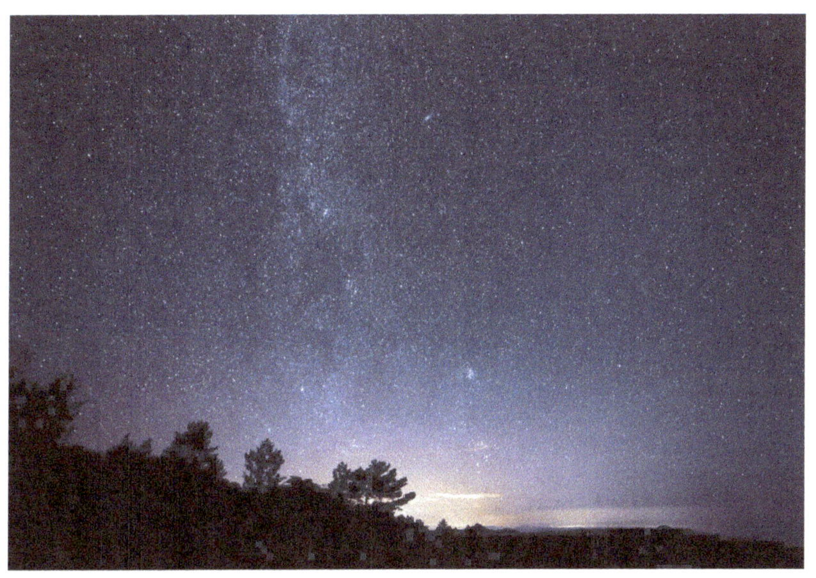

7

Earthing in Nature

Earthing, also known as grounding, is a way of connecting directly to the Earth's inherent energies which are an amazing source of well-being. The practice of earthing involves direct physical contact with the Earth, such as walking barefoot on grass, soil, or sand, swimming in natural bodies of water, or touching a tree. This simple yet powerful practice has historically been a natural aspect of human life but has largely been forgotten with our modern lifestyles. In this chapter, we will explore what earthing is, why it's important, and set the stage for how you can integrate this practice into your daily life for improved health and wellness.

The foundation of earthing lies in reconnecting with the Earth's electrons. Our planet possesses a natural, subtle electrical charge, and when you come into contact with it, these electrons are absorbed into your body. This process is akin to resetting your internal biological rhythm and facilitates various physiological processes—many people who practice earthing report immediate benefits like reduced stress, better sleep, and improved mood.

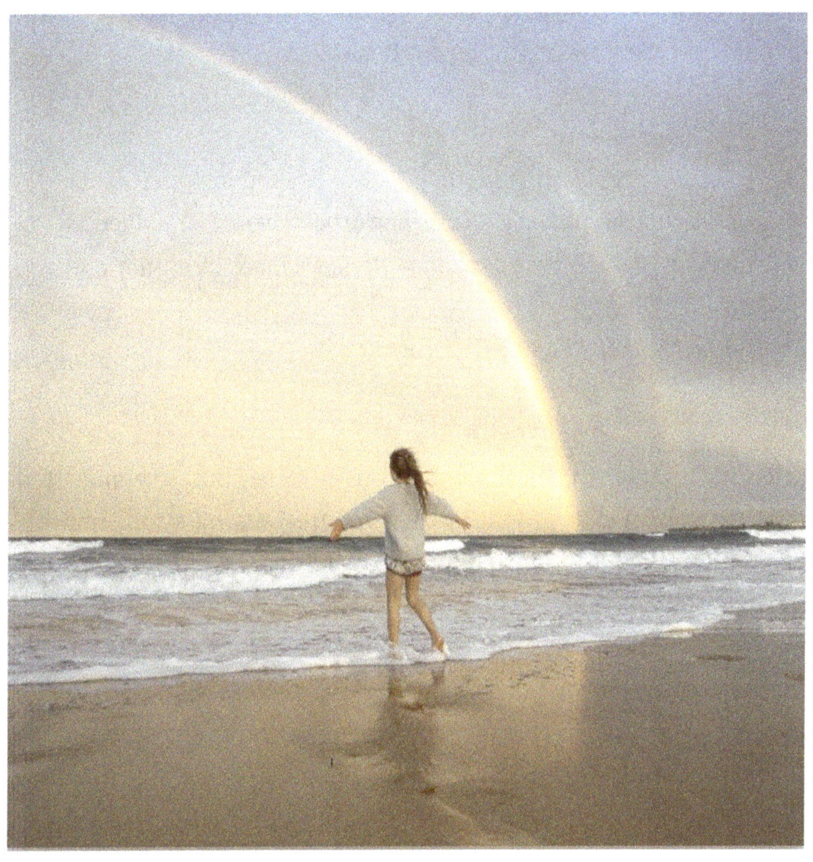

Earthing is not a new concept. For thousands of years, indigenous cultures around the world have recognized the importance of connecting with the Earth. Our ancestors maintained an intimate relationship with nature through spiritual rituals or everyday activities. This connection allowed them to live in harmony with the Earth, reaping its physical and mental benefits. In contrast, modern lifestyle trends have largely disconnected us from the natural world. We spend most of our time indoors, wearing insulating shoes and walking on artificial surfaces. This disconnect has led to a myriad of health concerns, from increased stress levels to chronic diseases. Earthing brings us back to nature, helping to restore and maintain our health.

"The old people came literally to love the soil and they sat or reclined on the ground with a feeling of being close to a mothering power. The soil was soothing, strengthening, cleansing and healing."
   Chief Luther Standing Bear (Ota Kte)

Scientific research increasingly supports the benefits of earthing. Studies have shown that grounding can reduce inflammation, improve heart rate variability, normalize cortisol levels (the body's primary stress hormone), and enhance overall well-being. For instance, a study published in the Journal of Environmental and Public Health in 2012 highlighted the many positive effects that grounding has on health, including improved sleep and reduced pain. While more research is still necessary to fully understand the mechanisms, the existing evidence is promising.

Earthing also promotes mindfulness and a deeper connection to the natural world. As you take the time to walk barefoot on the grass or sit by a lake, you become more present and attuned to the environment around you. This mindful interaction with nature can help reduce stress, re-centre your thoughts, and foster a sense of peace and tranquility. In today's fast-paced world, these moments of mindfulness are invaluable for maintaining mental health.

"It was good for the skin to touch the earth, and the old people liked to remove their moccasins and walk with bare feet on the sacred earth... the old Indian still sits upon the earth instead of propping himself up and away from its life-giving forces. For him, to sit or lie upon the ground is to be able to think more deeply and to feel more keenly. He can see more clearly into the mysteries of life and come closer in kinship to other lives about him."
Chief Luther Standing Bear (Ota Kte)

One of the main advantages of earthing is its simplicity. Unlike many wellness practices that require significant time, money, or specialized knowledge, earthing is accessible to everyone. All you need is a natural surface and a little bit of time. You don't have to buy expensive equipment or undergo complicated training. Just step outside, find a patch of earth and connect. Whether a few minutes a day or longer, every bit of time spent grounded adds significant health benefits.

Of course, earthing is also highly versatile. You can incorporate it into various activities and settings, from a morning meditation on the beach to an afternoon picnic in the park or an evening swim in a lake. It can be both a solitary practice and a social one, shared with friends and family. This flexibility makes it easy to adapt earthing to your lifestyle, no matter how busy or varied it might be.

I hope you feel empowered and inspired to make earthing a meaningful part of your life. Reconnecting with the Earth's natural energy can significantly impact your health, well-being, and overall quality of life, and it is so easy to do. You just need to spend a few minutes barefoot or touching a tree for the connection to work. Why not give it a try?

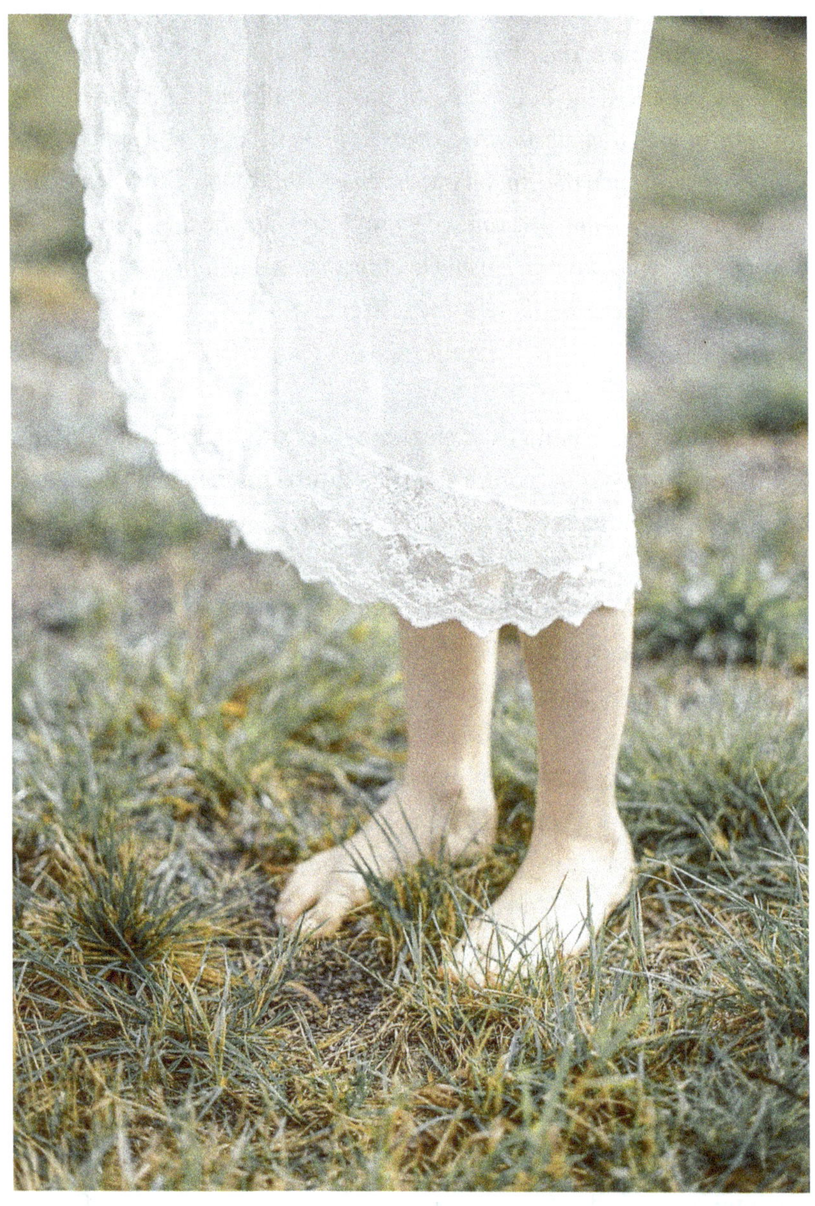

Please note: Medical and medication considerations.

Since earthing influences many basic physiological processes, if you are on medication for any condition, please consult your health care provider before you start, as you may need adjustment to your medication.

Reference:

Earthing Institute. (2023, October 12). *Medical and Medication Considerations - Earthing Institute.* https://earthinginstitute.net/medical-and-medication-considerations/

8

Animal-Assisted Ecotherapy

"What is man without the beasts? If all the beasts were gone, men would die from great loneliness of spirit, for whatever happens to the beasts also happens to man. All things are connected. Whatever befalls the earth befalls the children of the earth."
  -Chief Seattle

Benefits of Interacting with Animals.

Interacting with animals can help reduce stress, anxiety, and depression while boosting overall mood and happiness. Physical touch, for example, when petting or hugging a pet, releases oxytocin, a hormone associated with bonding and stress relief. Animals also encourage physical activity, whether taking a dog for a walk or birdwatching outdoors, contributing to better physical health. Furthermore, animals provide nonjudgmental companionship, offering emotional support and reducing loneliness.

Types of Animal-Assisted Therapy

Equine Therapy

Equine therapy involves interactions with horses, which can be particularly beneficial for people who have PTSD, anxiety, and developmental disorders. Grooming, feeding, and riding help improve emotional regulation, social skills, and physical strength. The bond between horse and human can be incredibly healing, fostering trust and empathy.

Canine Therapy

Dogs are known for their loyalty and unconditional love, making them excellent companions for therapeutic purposes. Canine therapy is commonly used in hospitals, nursing homes, and schools to help reduce stress and promote emotional well-being. Visiting therapy dogs can bring joy to patients, motivate physical rehabilitation, and even enhance children's reading skills by providing a nonjudgmental audience.

A study in the American Journal of Critical Care found that visits with therapy dogs improved cardiovascular health in heart patients, precipitating lowered blood pressure and stress hormone levels.

Feline Therapy

Cats may not be as active as dogs, but their calming presence can provide significant emotional support. Feline therapy is particularly beneficial for people with high stress levels and anxiety. The simple act of petting a cat can lower blood pressure and create a zen-like atmosphere, making it easier to relax and reflect.

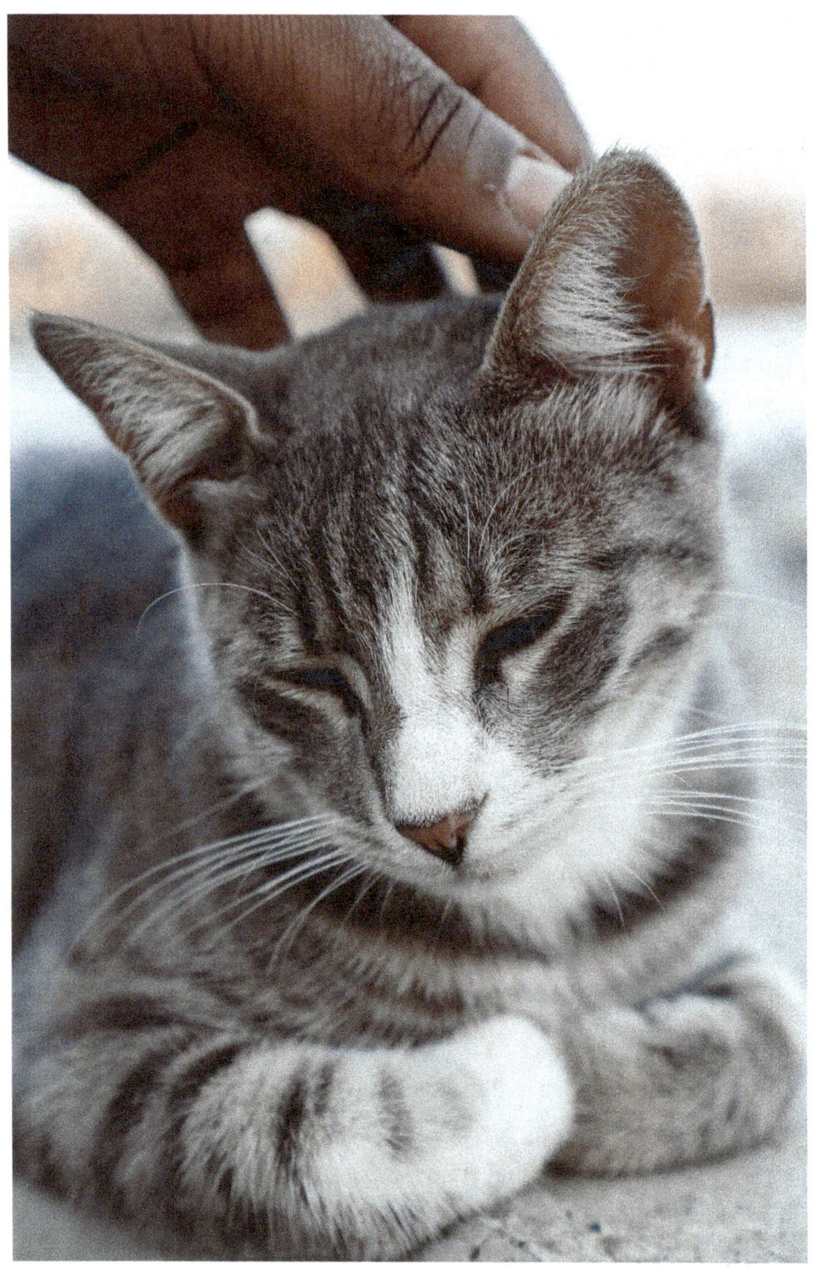

Farm Animal Therapy

Interacting with farm animals like goats, sheep, and chickens can be a fun and therapeutic experience. Farm animal therapy often involves caring for and feeding the animals, which can be grounding and offer a sense of purpose. This type of therapy is especially beneficial for children and individuals with developmental disabilities, helping to improve social skills, teamwork, and self-esteem.

Bird Watching

Birds are all around us just waiting to be noticed. Be a "birder" and explore the bird life in your vicinity! Seeing and hearing birds can significantly improve mental health. According to a Scientific Reports(2022) study, encounters with birdlife were associated with lasting improvements in mental well-being. These improvements were evident not only in healthy people but also in those with a diagnosis of depression.

Success Stories and Practical Tips

Countless success stories back the transformative power of animal-assisted ecotherapy. For instance, veterans with PTSD have shown remarkable improvement in symptoms such as anxiety, flashbacks, and nightmares after engaging in equine therapy. Seniors in nursing homes have experienced reduced loneliness and improved cognitive function after regular visits from therapy dogs. Even stressed-out college students have reported feeling more relaxed and focused after spending time with therapy cats during finals week.

If you're interested in integrating animal-assisted ecotherapy into your life, you could begin with observation of wildlife, such as bird watching.

Bird watching is an easy and fascinating hobby to take up wherever you live. You could start by setting up a bird feeder outside your window to attract birds, which you can then observe close-up. Venturing out to a nearby park, garden or just the trees along your street, you will surely notice a few species of birds if you keep your eyes peeled. Listening to these birds' songs and observing them is the start of a wonderful relationship with our feathered friends.

Next, you may wish to identify and name the birds you encounter and perhaps keep a journal, recording your experiences. For more information on Birding, including guides and apps that help with identification, you may visit:

https://birda.org

or

https://www.audubon.org/birding/how-to-start-birding.

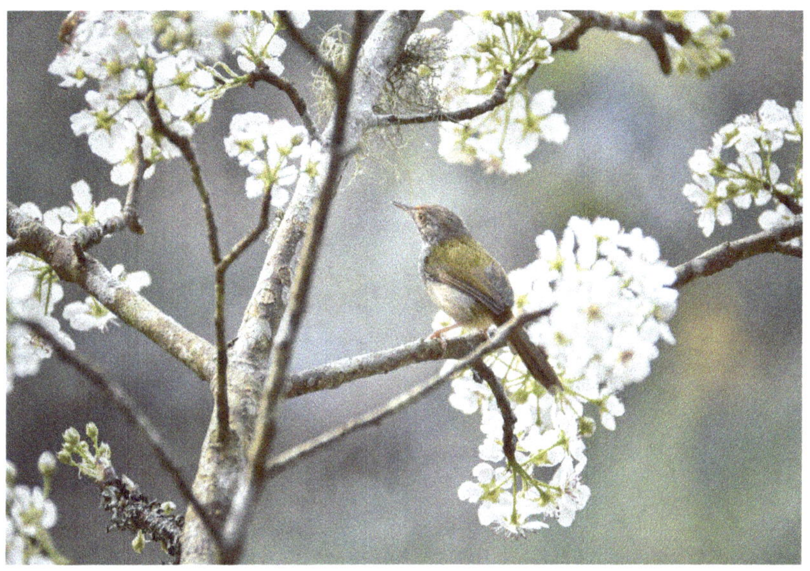

For a more tactile approach, you could visit a local animal shelter or volunteer to walk dogs. If practical, consider adopting a pet to bring unconditional love and companionship into your everyday life. Many organizations also offer structured animal-assisted therapy programs that you can join.

Ultimately, the goal is to find a form of animal interaction that resonates with you and fits into your lifestyle. By doing so, you can tap into the endless benefits our furry, feathered, or even scaly friends offer, enriching your life with joy, purpose, and well-being.

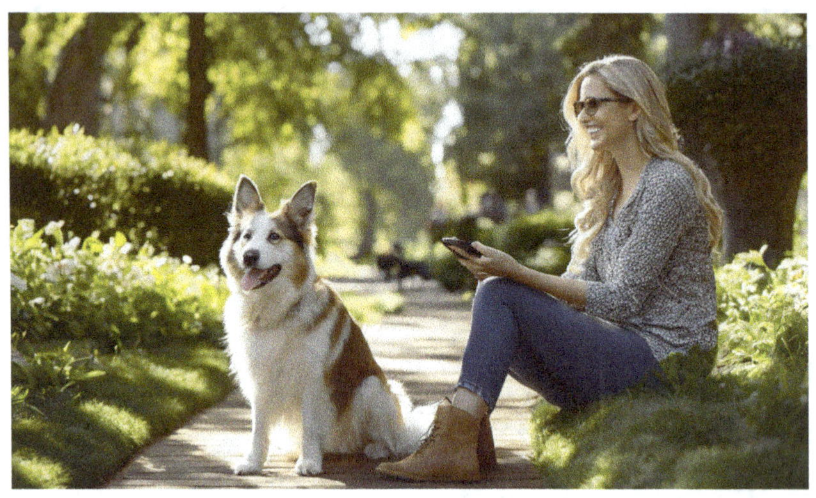

9

Adventure and Wilderness Therapy

Adventure and wilderness therapy is a unique and powerful form of ecotherapy that combines the physical challenge of outdoor activities with the mental and emotional benefits of being in natural settings. This therapy approach emphasizes personal growth, self-discovery, and emotional healing through direct engagement with the wilderness.

Adventure and wilderness therapy generally involves a guided experience in a natural environment. Participants might find themselves hiking up a mountain, navigating through a forest, or camping under the stars. These activities aren't just about physical exercise; they're carefully designed to push boundaries and encourage self-reflection. The wilderness can act as both a mirror and a catalyst for personal growth. The challenges faced outdoors—a steep climb, unpredictable weather, or simply the sheer vastness of nature—can parallel the personal struggles one faces daily, providing insights into resilience, problem-solving, and self-efficacy.

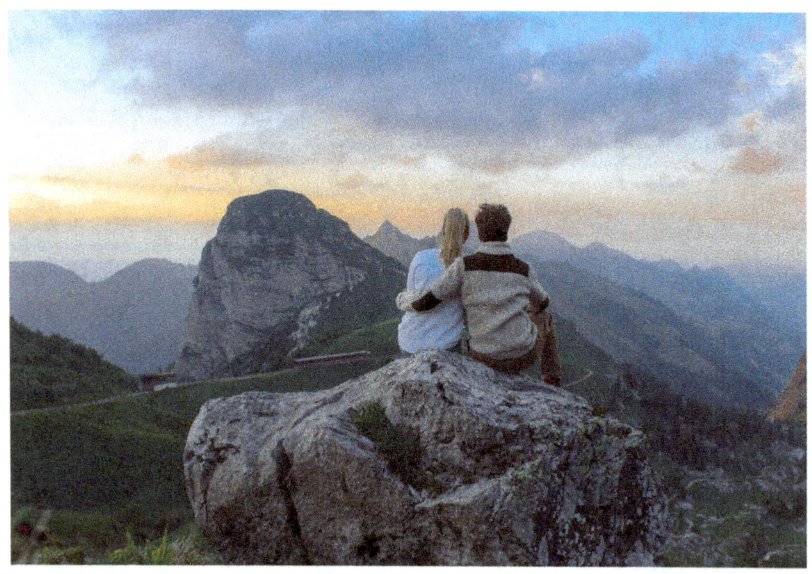

One key benefit of adventure and wilderness therapy is the sense of accomplishment and empowerment it fosters. Successfully completing a challenging hike or setting up a campsite can significantly boost self-confidence. These achievements, no matter how small, can lead to a greater sense of self-worth and a more positive self-image. For individuals dealing with issues such as depression, anxiety, or low self-esteem, these experiences can be transformative.

Moreover, being surrounded by nature has inherent therapeutic benefits. Research shows that spending time in natural environments can reduce stress, lower blood pressure, and improve overall mood. The sights, sounds, and smells of the wilderness—a babbling brook, the rustling of leaves, the scent of pine—create a calming sensory experience that soothes the mind and body. The physical activity involved in adventure therapy also releases endorphins, the body's natural mood elevators, thus contributing to overall emotional well-being.

Another essential element of wilderness therapy is the opportunity for introspection and connection. The solitude and stillness of natural settings can facilitate deep self-reflection, allowing individuals to connect with their inner thoughts and emotions. Therapy professionals who accompany participants can guide this reflection and offer support through the process. Group settings also provide a unique form of social interaction, where participants can bond over shared experiences and provide mutual support, fostering a sense of community and belonging.

Many established wilderness therapy programs are available worldwide, offering structured experiences led by trained professionals. These programs often target specific populations, such as troubled teens, individuals with substance abuse issues, or people looking for personal development. One example is Outward Bound, an organization that uses challenging expeditions in the wilderness to teach valuable life skills and foster personal growth. Participants in these programs often report significant improvements in their self-esteem, coping skills, and overall mental health.

However, you don't need to join a formal program to benefit from wilderness therapy. Simple activities such as a hike, a weekend camping trip, or even a day spent exploring a nature reserve can have similar therapeutic effects. The key is to engage with nature in a meaningful way, allowing yourself to be fully present and open to the experiences it offers. Whether you're tackling a challenging trail or simply sitting quietly by a lake, the wilderness has the power to heal, inspire, and transform.

Embrace the adventure, challenge yourself, and let the natural world guide you on a journey of healing and self-discovery.

52

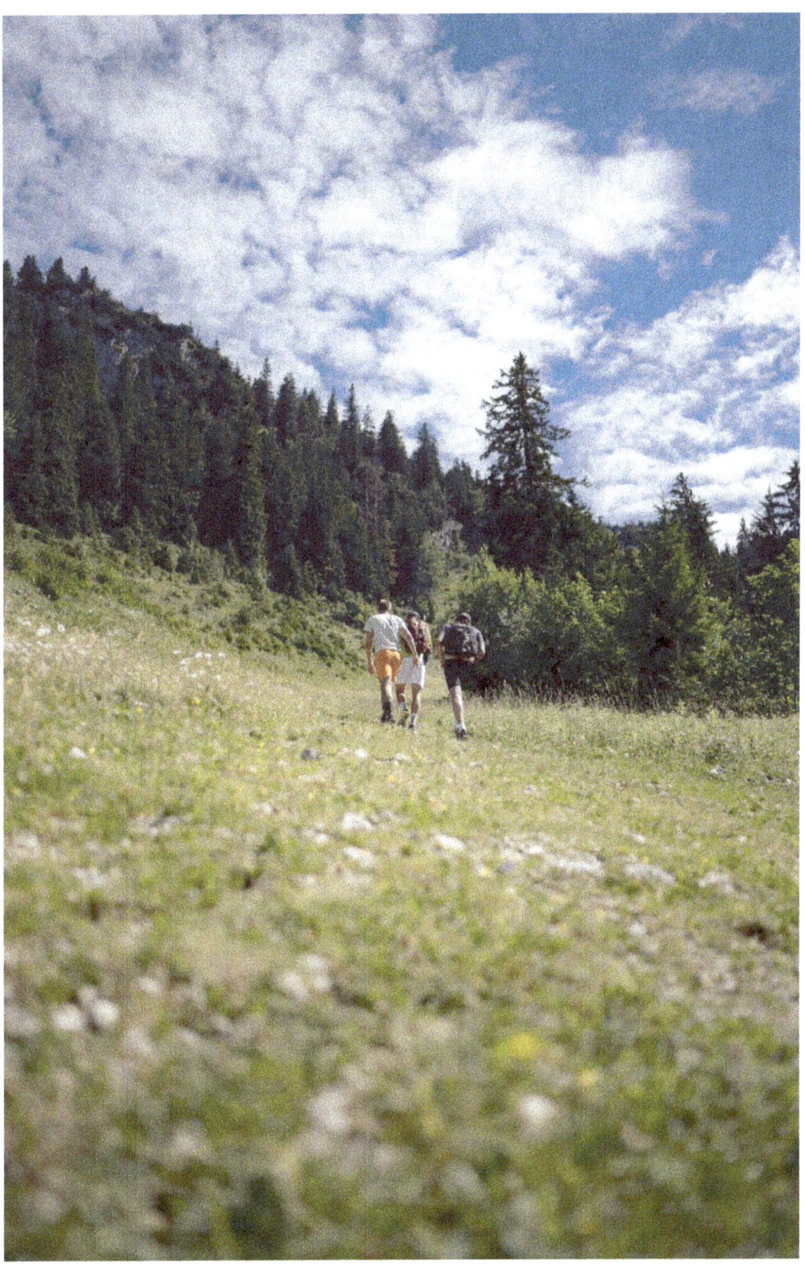

Safety Note

There are obvious dangers to be aware of in the wild: dangerous terrain, wild animals, poisonous plants and biting insects that you may come across as well as bad weather so it pays to be prepared.

Be Prepared

- Research the trail, get advice from authorities and check the weather forecast.
- Wear suitable clothing and footwear and use insecticide.
- Protect yourself from the sun and rain with a hat and raincoat.
- Stay hydrated: Bring enough water, or a method of purifying it, and provisions.
- Bring a first aid kit with bandages, antiseptic and painkillers.
- Keep to designated pathways.
- Always inform someone about your destination and intended time of return so they can contact authorities in case of emergency.
- what3words is an app that helps anyone find a location anywhere in the world using 3 words. It can help emergency services find your precise location.

Be responsible and safe!

10

Creating Your Own Ecotherapy Practice

Creating your own ecotherapy practice doesn't have to be complex or time-consuming. The beauty of ecotherapy lies in its simplicity and accessibility. You can start small and gradually build a routine that suits your lifestyle and needs. Let's look at some easy steps to incorporate ecotherapy into your daily life and find your unique connection with nature.

Start With Observation

The first step towards embracing ecotherapy is to begin observing your surroundings. Take a moment each day to notice the natural elements around you: the trees lining your street, a local park, or a small garden. Pay attention to the details. What kind of plants and animals do you see? How do the changes in weather affect the environment? These small observations help you cultivate mindfulness and deepen your connection with nature.

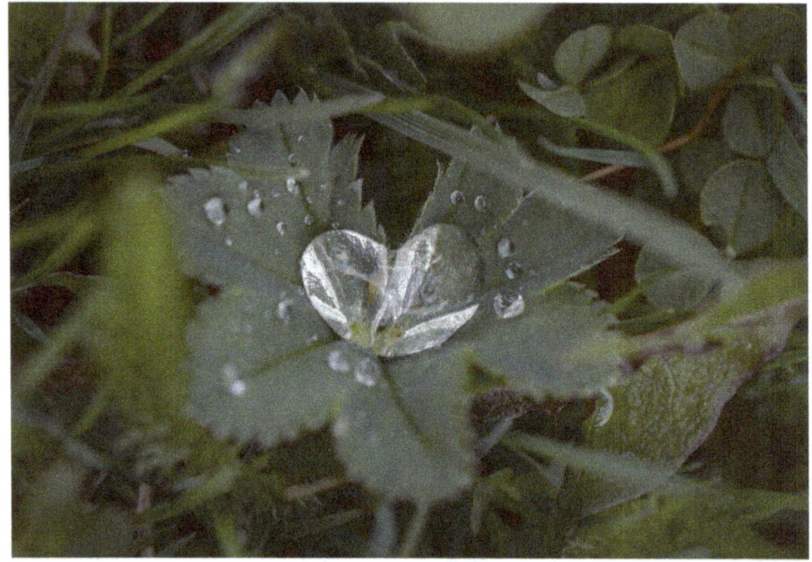

Make Time for Green Spaces

You don't need to venture far to experience the benefits of nature. Make it a habit to spend time in nearby parks or gardens. Even a short walk can significantly impact your mental and physical well-being. Try to identify a few green spaces near your home or work and visit them regularly. Over time, you'll start to notice how these visits improve your mood and energy levels.

Engage in Simple Activities

Engaging in simple activities such as earthing, walking, jogging, or meditating in nature can be incredibly therapeutic. Moving your body outdoors, surrounded by nature is a powerful form of ecotherapy. If possible, incorporate these activities into your daily routine. For example, consider walking or biking to work instead of driving. These small changes can make a big difference in how connected you feel to nature.

Bring Nature Indoors

If you find it challenging to spend time outdoors, consider bringing nature indoors. Houseplants, flowers, and even images of natural landscapes can have calming effects. Create a mini garden on your balcony, or place a few potted plants around your home. Studies show that simply looking at pictures of nature can reduce stress and improve mental health!

Mindful Eating and Drinking

Another way to connect with nature is through mindful eating and drinking. Focus on consuming organic and locally sourced foods. Pay attention to the flavours, textures, and origins of your food. This practice enhances your connection to the environment and promotes a healthier lifestyle.

Practice Forest Bathing

If you have access to a forest or wooded area, practice 'Shinrin-yoku' or forest bathing. This Japanese practice involves immersing yourself in the forest atmosphere and mindfully absorbing the sights, sounds, and scents. You don't need to hike or do strenuous exercise. Just being present in the forest and taking in the surroundings can profoundly affect your mental state.

Connect with Water

Similarly, spending time near bodies of water can be incredibly soothing. Whether it's a river, lake, or ocean, water has a unique way of calming the mind. If you have the opportunity, incorporate water-based activities such as swimming, kayaking, or simply sitting by the water into your routine.

Even your daily shower can be a refreshing preparation or a welcome respite to your busy day, especially with intention and the recognition you now have of its benefits!

Animal Companionship

Animals can also play a significant role in your ecotherapy practice. Whether you have pets or enjoy birdwatching, engaging with animals can elevate your mood and reduce feelings of loneliness. Consider volunteering at an animal shelter or spending time with pets in a natural setting.

Create a Personal Sanctuary

Finally, create your personal nature sanctuary. It could be a quiet corner of your garden, a cozy balcony space, or even a room in your house dedicated to relaxation and mindfulness. Fill this space with natural elements that bring you peace and joy. Use this sanctuary for meditation, reading, or simply unwinding after a long day.

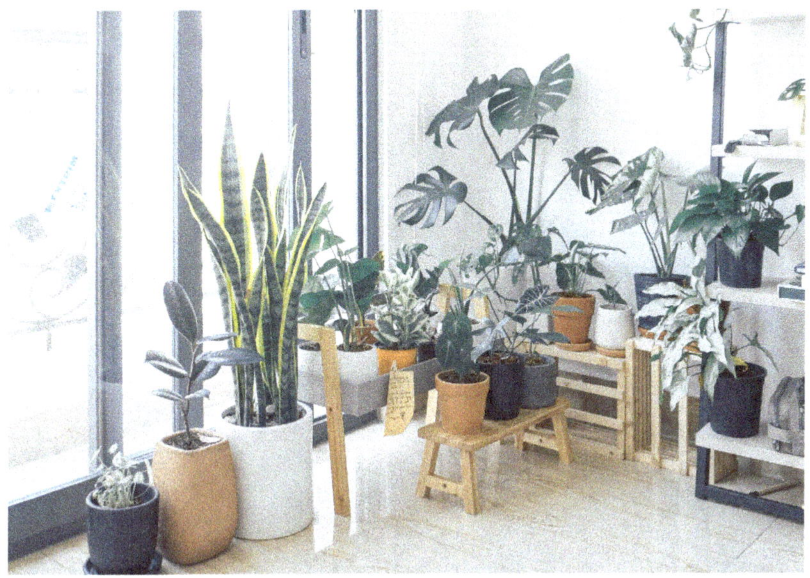

In conclusion, integrating ecotherapy into your daily life is about creating intentional moments to connect with nature. By starting small and building a routine that fits your lifestyle, you can experience the profound benefits of this practice.

11

Respect for Nature: A Call for Mindful Stewardship of the Earth

As we step into the wild, we are reminded of the intricate web of life that surrounds us. The rustle of leaves, the whisper of the wind, and the distant call of a bird all serve as a gentle reminder that we are merely visitors in this vast, interconnected ecosystem. In our quest for solace and healing through ecotherapy, it is imperative that we cultivate a deep respect for nature, understanding that our actions have far-reaching consequences, both for ourselves and for the generations that will follow.

"We will be known forever by the tracks we leave." - Dakota Tribe

The Philosophy of Minimal Impact

When we venture into nature, it is crucial to Leave No Trace -to take only what we need and leave the place as we find it. Each step we take should reflect our commitment to preserving the beauty around us. Collecting souvenirs—a rock, a flower, or even a feather—may seem innocuous.

However, it disrupts the natural order and deprives others of the joy of experiencing these wonders. Instead, we should immerse ourselves in the moment, allowing nature's sights, sounds, and scents to etch themselves into our minds, creating lasting memories that need no physical token.

"Take only memories, leave nothing but footprints", Chief Seattle, *Chief of the Suquamish and Duwamish tribes.*

The Legacy of Our Actions

As we navigate through forests, mountains, and waterways, we must confront the reality of the damage we have inflicted upon our planet. From deforestation to pollution, our collective actions have left scars on the Earth that may never fully heal. Climate change, habitat destruction, and species extinction are urgent reminders of our responsibility to safeguard the environment. The beauty of nature is not just for our enjoyment; it is vital for the survival of countless species, including our own.

To honour the legacy of those who came before us and to protect the world for future generations, we must commit to a paradigm shift in our relationship with nature. This means embracing sustainable practices, advocating for conservation efforts, and recognizing that every small action counts. Whether it's picking up litter during a hike, using eco-friendly products, or supporting organizations dedicated to environmental preservation, we can all contribute to the healing of our planet.

A Shared Existence

We are not separate from nature; we are a part of it. Our well-being is inextricably linked to the health of the ecosystems that sustain us. Clean air, fresh water, fertile soil, and biodiversity are not just resources; they are the very foundations of life. By fostering a sense of connection with the natural world, we can begin to appreciate its value beyond just what it provides. This shift in perspective allows us to see ourselves as caretakers of the environment, embracing the responsibility of looking after our Earth.

In our pursuit of ecotherapy, let us remember that nature is not a backdrop for our human experiences but a vibrant, living entity deserving of our respect and protection. Each time we enter the wild, let us enter with humility and gratitude, recognizing the privilege of being part of this magnificent world.

Creating a Culture of Respect

To cultivate respect for nature, we must also educate ourselves and others about the importance of biodiversity and ecological balance. Sharing knowledge about local flora and fauna, participating in community clean-ups, and engaging in discussions about environmental issues can foster a culture of respect and stewardship. Understanding the intricate relationships within ecosystems makes us more mindful of our impact and more motivated to protect the natural world.

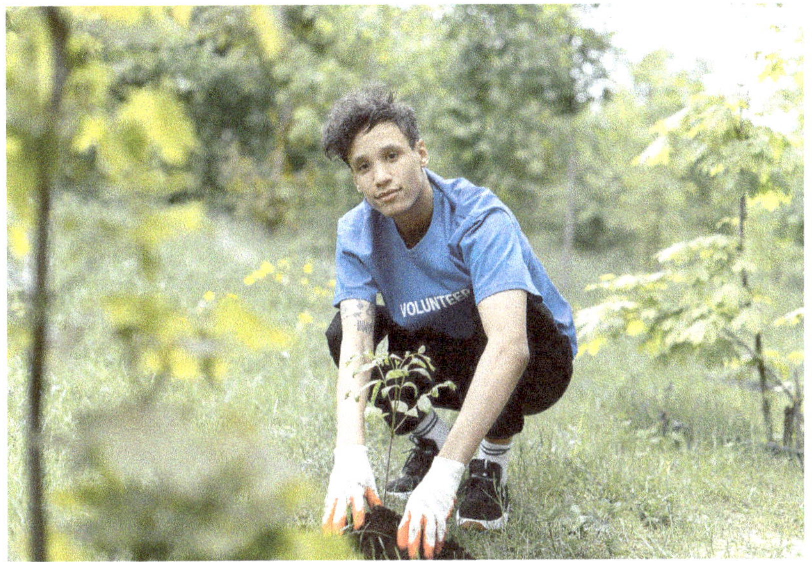

Photo by Mikhail Nilov

Conclusion: A Call to Action

Our time in the wild is not only a chance to heal and rejuvenate but also an opportunity to reflect on our role as caretakers of this planet. By leaving no trace, cherishing our experiences, and advocating for the environment, we can ensure that the beauty of nature endures for generations to come.

Let us walk gently upon the Earth, honouring the gifts it provides, and commit ourselves to nurturing the world that nurtures us. In doing so, we not only enrich our own lives but also pave the way for a future where both humanity and nature can thrive in harmony.

"May the sun bring you new energy by day. May the moon softly restore you by night. May the rain wash away your worries. May the breeze blow new strength into your being. May you walk gently through the world and know its beauty all the days of your life."
  Apache blessing

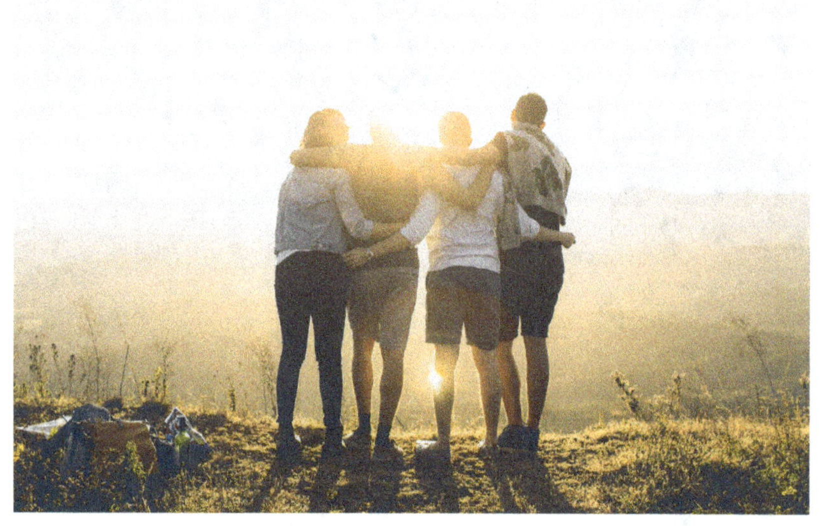

References

Animal-Assisted therapy research. (n.d.). UCLA Health. https://www.ucla health.org/programs/pac/about-us/animal-assisted-therapy-researc h

Asher, H. (2023a, June 18). *The Origins of Forest Bathing — an Darach Forest therapy.* An Darach Forest Therapy. https://silvotherapy.co.uk/ articles/the-origins-of-forest-bathing

Asher, H. (2023b, November 18). *The benefits of hugging trees — an Darach forest therapy.* An Darach Forest Therapy. https://silvotherapy.co.uk/art icles/benefits-of-hugging-trees#:~:text=Studies%20show%20that% 20after%20people,of%20wellbeing%2C%20calmness%20and%20tru st.

Atchley, R. A., Strayer, D. L., & Atchley, P. (2012). Creativity in the Wild: Improving Creative Reasoning through Immersion in Natural Settings. *PLoS ONE, 7*(12), e51474. https://doi.org/10.1371/journal.pone.0051474

Azeemi, S. T. Y., & Raza, M. (2000). A critical analysis of chromotherapy and its scientific evolution. *Evidence-based Complementary and Alternative Medicine, 2*(4), 481–488. https://doi.org/10.1093/ecam/neh137

Being in natural light improves mood, increases happiness. (2022, March 25). UCLA Health. https://www.uclahealth.org/news/article/being-in-natural-light-improves-mood-increases-happiness

Birding. (n.d.). Audubon. https://www.audubon.org/birding

BlockBlueLight UK. (2020, June 1). The incredible benefits of Red & Infrared Light therapy - How the right light therapy device can help you. *BlockBlueLight UK.* https://www.blockbluelight.co.uk/blogs/news/benefits-of-red-light-therapy#:~:text=It%20strengthens%20the%20anti%2Dinflammatory,to%20cells%20throughout%20the%20body.

Bratman, G. N., Hamilton, J. P., Hahn, K. S., Daily, G. C., & Gross, J. J. (2015). Nature experience reduces rumination and subgenual prefrontal cortex activation. *Proceedings of the National Academy of Sciences, 112*(28), 8567–8572. https://doi.org/10.1073/pnas.1510459112

Britton, E., Kindermann, G., Domegan, C., & Carlin, C. (2018). Blue care: a systematic review of blue space interventions for health and wellbeing. *Health Promotion International, 35*(1), 50–69. https://doi.org/10.1093/heapro/day103

Burns, A. C., Saxena, R., Vetter, C., Phillips, A. J. K., Lane, J. M., & Cain, S. W. (2021). Time spent in outdoor light is associated with mood, sleep, and circadian rhythm-related outcomes: A cross-sectional and longitudinal study in over 400,000 UK Biobank participants. *Journal of Affective Disorders, 295,* 347–352. https://doi.org/10.1016/j.jad.2021.08.056

Chevalier, G., Sinatra, S. T., Oschman, J. L., Sokal, K., & Sokal, P. (2012). Earthing: health implications of reconnecting the human body to the Earth's surface electrons. *Journal of Environmental and Public Health*, 2012, 1–8. https://doi.org/10.1155/2012/291541

Colour therapy information. (n.d.). Colour Therapy Healing. https://www.colourtherapyhealing.com/

Coss, R. G., & Keller, C. M. (2022). Transient decreases in blood pressure and heart rate with increased subjective level of relaxation while viewing water compared with adjacent ground. *Journal of Environmental Psychology, 81*, 101794. https://doi.org/10.1016/j.jenvp.2022.101794

Coventry, P. A., Brown, J., Pervin, J., Brabyn, S., Pateman, R., Breedvelt, J., Gilbody, S., Stancliffe, R., McEachan, R., & White, P. (2021). Nature-based outdoor activities for mental and physical health: Systematic review and meta-analysis. *SSM - Population Health, 16*, 100934. https://doi.org/10.1016/j.ssmph.2021.100934

David. (2024, February 9). Red light therapy for neurological conditions explained. *Occupational Therapy Brisbane.* https://occupationaltherapybrisbane.com.au/red-light-therapy-for-neurological-conditions-explained/#:~:text=Red%20light%20therapy%20works%20by,rich%20blood%20to%20the%20brain.

DrLaPuma, & DrLaPuma. (2021, January 31). *What is Blue Care? | Healthy Living, Wellness & Nutrition Expert | Dr John La Puma.* Dr John La Puma | Wellness and Nutrition Expert. https://www.drjohnlapuma.com/wellness-and-health/what-is-blue-care/

Earthing Institute. (2021, February 22). *What is Earthing - Earthing*

Institute. https://earthinginstitute.net/what-is-earthing/

Earthing Institute. (2023, October 12). *Medical and Medication Consid-erations - Earthing Institute.* https://earthinginstitute.net/medical-and-medication-considerations/

Featured news - Green spaces deliver lasting mental health benefits - University of Exeter. (n.d.). University of Exeter. https://news-archiv e.exeter.ac.uk/featurednews/title_349054_en.html

Hamblin, M. R. (2016). Shining light on the head: Photobiomodulation for brain disorders. *BBA Clinical, 6,* 113–124. https://doi.org/10.1016/ j.bbacli.2016.09.002

Home. (n.d.). Husson University. https://www.husson.edu/online/blog/ 2022/07/benefits-of-animal-assisted-therapy

Jbysdev, & Jbysdev. (2023, October 10). *How being near water improves your mood | JBYS.* Jefferson Beach Yacht Sales. https://jbys.com/water-improves-your-mood/

Neumann, K. D. (2024, January 12). Red light therapy: benefits, side effects and uses. *Forbes Health.* https://www.forbes.com/health/wellne ss/red-light-therapy/

Nichols, W. J. (22 C.E.). *Blue mind: The surprising science that shows how being near, in, on, or under water can make you happier, healthier, more connected, and better at what you do* [Kindle]. Little, Brown. (Original work published 2014)

Nurturing nature: The therapeutic benefits of gardening. (2024, February

13). University Canada West (UCW). https://www.ucanwest.ca/blog/life style-culture/nurturing-nature-the-therapeutic-benefits-of-garden ing/

Ohwovoriole, T. (2024, January 12). *Color therapy types, techniques, and benefits*. Verywell Mind. https://www.verywellmind.com/color-therap y-definition-types-techniques-and-efficacy-5194910

Smalley, A. J., & White, M. P. (2023). Beyond blue-sky thinking: Diurnal patterns and ephemeral meteorological phenomena impact appraisals of beauty, awe, and value in urban and natural landscapes. *Journal of Environmental Psychology, 86*, 101955. https://doi.org/10.1016/j.jenvp.2 023.101955

Van Den Berg, M., Maas, J., Muller, R., Braun, A., Kaandorp, W., Van Lien, R., Van Poppel, M., Van Mechelen, W., & Van Den Berg, A. (2015). Autonomic nervous system responses to viewing green and built settings: differentiating between sympathetic and parasympathetic activity. *International Journal of Environmental Research and Public Health, 12*(12), 15860–15874. https://doi.org/10.3390/ijerph121215026

We should all be watching more sunsets for the good of our mental health: new study. (2023, April 21). Nationalpost. https://nationalpost.com/ health/mental-health-research-sunsets

White, J. (2024, September 4). *Birda | a global birdwatching app to connect with nature*. Birda. https://birda.org/

White, M. P., Alcock, I., Grellier, J., Wheeler, B. W., Hartig, T., Warber, S. L., Bone, A., Depledge, M. H., & Fleming, L. E. (2019). Spending at least 120 minutes a week in nature is associated with good health and wellbeing. *Scientific Reports*, 9(1). https://doi.org/10.1038/s41598-019-44097-3

Why are forests so important for life on Earth? · Planet Wild. (2024, February 28). https://planetwild.com/blog/why-are-forests-important

Zhao, Y., Bao, W., Yang, B., Liang, J., Gui, Z., Huang, S., Chen, Y., Dong, G., & Chen, Y. (2022). Association between greenspace and blood pressure: A systematic review and meta-analysis. *The Science of the Total Environment*, 817, 152513. https://doi.org/10.1016/j.scitotenv.2021.152513